AF430003

# SIBO Diet

## A Beginner's Step-by-Step Guide To Reversing SIBO Symptoms Through Diet with Selected Recipes

BRANDON GILTA

All rights reserved No part of this book may be reproduced, or stored in a retrieval system, or transmitted in any form or by any means, electronic, mechanical, photocopying, recording, or otherwise, without express written permission of the publisher.

Copyright © 2019 Brandon Gilta

All rights reserved.

# Disclaimer

By reading this disclaimer, you are accepting the terms of the disclaimer in full. If you disagree with this disclaimer, please do not read the guide.

All of the content within this guide is provided for informational and educational purposes only, and should not be accepted as independent medical or other professional advice. The author is not a doctor, physician, nurse, mental health provider, or registered nutritionist/dietician. Therefore, using and reading this guide does not establish any form of a physician-patient relationship.

Always consult with a physician or another qualified health provider with any issues or questions you might have regarding any sort of medical condition. Do not ever disregard any qualified professional medical advice or delay seeking that advice because of anything you have read in this guide. The information in this guide is not intended to be any sort of medical advice and should not be used in lieu of any medical advice by a licensed and qualified medical professional.

The information in this guide has been compiled from a variety of known sources. However, the author cannot attest to or guarantee the accuracy of each source and thus should not be held liable for any errors or omissions.

You acknowledge that the publisher of this guide will not be held liable for any loss or damage of any kind incurred as a result of this guide or the reliance on any information provided within this guide. You acknowledge and agree that you assume all risk and responsibility for any action you undertake in response to the information in this guide.

Using this guide does not guarantee any particular result (e.g., weight loss or a cure). By reading this guide, you acknowledge that there are no guarantees to any specific outcome or results you can expect.

All product names, diet plans, or names used in this guide are for identification purposes only and are the property of their respective owners. The use of these names does not imply endorsement. All other trademarks cited herein are the property of their respective owners.

Where applicable, this guide is not intended to be a substitute for the original work of this diet plan and is, at most, a supplement to the original work for this diet plan and never a direct substitute. This guide is a personal expression of the facts of that diet plan.

Where applicable, persons shown in the cover images are stock photography models and the publisher has obtained the rights to use the images through license agreements with third-party stock image companies.

# Introduction

Small Intestinal Bacterial Overgrowth (SIBO) is a common digestive disorder that occurs when there is excessive growth of bacteria in the small intestine. SIBO can lead to a wide range of unpleasant symptoms, including bloating, abdominal pain, and diarrhea or constipation. If left untreated, it can also cause long-term damage to the digestive system.

Thankfully, a SIBO-specific diet can help alleviate the symptoms of this condition. The SIBO diet works by removing or limiting certain types of food that can fuel the overgrowth of bacteria in the small intestine. By minimizing the number of fermentable carbohydrates consumed, SIBO patients can effectively starve the bacteria and improve their digestive health.

On the other hand, a SIBO-friendly diet should include foods that are low in FODMAP and easy to digest. Some examples of suitable foods include meat, fish, eggs, low-FODMAP vegetables such as carrots and spinach, and gluten-free grains like quinoa and rice. It's also recommended to eat foods that are high in fiber to help promote healthy gut function.

While a SIBO diet can be an effective way to manage the symptoms of this condition, it's important to work with a healthcare professional to develop a personalized treatment plan. This will help to ensure a balanced and nutritious diet that is tailored to each individual's specific needs.

In this guide, we will talk about the following:

- Small Intestinal Bacterial Growth (SIBO)
- SIBO Symptoms and treatments
- The SIBO Diet
- Benefits and Disadvantages of the SIBO Diet
- Sample Meal Plan and Recipes

So, without further ado, let's dive right into the world of SIBO and learn all about it!

# Table of Contents

# THE SMALL INTESTINAL BACTERIAL GROWTH (SIBO)

We all have beneficial bacteria in our stomach that helps with digestion and allows the production of the right amount of gastric acid in our small intestines. They also help fight the bad bacteria in the food we eat. The bacteria in the small intestine are different from those in the large intestine, and each has different functions.

When there is excessive growth of bacteria in the small intestines or if the bacteria present in that area are replaced by the kind of bacteria found in the large intestine, it results in SIBO. It is a combination of various bacteria types, not just one. These bacterial colonies can cause a range of health issues, from bloating to malabsorption. The human small intestine is usually sterile, so SIBO can take a toll on our overall well-being.

Many cases of SIBO are found to be an overgrowth of bacteria that are supposed to be in the colon but are found in the small bowel, and there are only rare cases of an overgrowth of bacteria in the small bowel itself. Overgrown bacteria are found in the lower part of the small intestine.

Food that is difficult for the higher part of the small intestine to digest travels to the lower part, where the overgrown bacteria eat it. The food serves as fuel for the bacteria instead of becoming a nutrient for the body.

When the bacteria consume the food, they ferment it and produce gasses that result in bloating, burping, or gas release. Because the body does not get the nutrients it needs from food, instead of getting healthy, the person will suffer from many more diseases.

SIBO is not contagious, unlike other gastrointestinal diseases. SIBO is often neglected because a person might be suffering from abdominal pain and the doctors will not be able to see anything wrong with his or her body, especially when the person does not suffer from any other diseases.

The doctors will see the body as normal because, in its normal state, the intestines already contain bacteria. SIBO will only be diagnosed as it is once the doctor considers the possibility of SIBO and performs tests precisely for SIBO.

**Symptoms of SIBO**

**Bloating**

Small intestinal bacterial overgrowth (SIBO) can cause a range of symptoms, but bloating is one of the most common. When there is an overgrowth of bacteria in the small intestine, they can produce excessive amounts of gas, leading to a feeling of fullness, hardness, or swelling in the stomach.

## Abdominal pain

Small intestinal bacterial overgrowth (SIBO) brings with it a range of symptoms, one of the most prominent being abdominal pain. This pain can vary in intensity from mild discomfort to debilitating agony and may be continuous or intermittent.

According to theory, the main causes of the pain are gas buildup and bacterial overgrowth-induced intestinal lining inflammation. Interestingly, some studies suggest that up to 80% of IBS patients also suffer from SIBO, further tying the condition to a host of debilitating digestive symptoms.

## Diarrhea or constipation

SIBO, or small intestinal bacterial overgrowth, can lead to both diarrhea and constipation, two contrasting symptoms that can disrupt one's daily routine. Frequent urges to go to the bathroom or the inability to have a bowel movement can lead to discomfort and frustration.

This occurs due to an imbalance in the gut bacteria, leading to difficulty digesting and processing food. It is important to seek medical attention if experiencing such symptoms, as SIBO can have adverse effects on nutrient absorption and overall health if left untreated.

## Nausea and vomiting

Small Intestinal Bacterial Overgrowth (SIBO) is a gastrointestinal disorder that results from the excessive growth of bacteria in the small intestine. The overgrowth of harmful bacteria that can result in infection is one of the common symptoms of SIBO, along with nausea and vomiting.

The bacterial overgrowth inhibits proper digestion and nutrient absorption, which can result in gastrointestinal issues such as bloating, gas, and diarrhea, in addition to nausea and vomiting. While these symptoms may be mild at first, if left untreated, they can progress and lead to adverse health outcomes. Early detection and treatment of SIBO are crucial to alleviate symptoms and prevent subsequent complications.

**Fatigue**

SIBO, or small intestinal bacterial overgrowth, can wreak havoc on the body's energy levels, leaving individuals feeling completely drained and fatigued. This is because the overgrowth of bacteria in the small intestine can lead to a reduction in nutrient absorption, particularly vitamins, and minerals that are necessary for cellular energy production.

Furthermore, the presence of excess bacteria can cause inflammation throughout the body, increasing stress on the immune system and further exacerbating fatigue. While physical activity can certainly contribute to feelings of tiredness, the fatigue associated with SIBO is more pervasive and persistent, often leaving individuals feeling depleted and unable to tackle even the simplest of tasks.

It's important to consult with a healthcare professional if you're experiencing chronic fatigue, as there may be an underlying cause such as SIBO that requires medical attention.

## Joint pain

In addition to digestive symptoms, individuals with small intestinal bacterial overgrowth (SIBO) may also experience joint pain. This occurs as a result of inflammation in the gut, which can trigger an immune response that leads to joint discomfort.

The relationship between SIBO and joint pain is not fully understood, but it is believed that the bacteria in the gut may release inflammatory substances that travel throughout the body and contribute to joint inflammation.

## Skin problems

Skin problems such as rashes or eczema can be indicative of small intestinal bacterial overgrowth (SIBO). The bacteria present in your gut can produce toxins that not only affect your gastrointestinal health but also your overall well-being.

These toxins can lead to harmful inflammation, causing symptoms such as skin rash or eczema. To mitigate this, it's imperative to address the underlying cause of the digestive issue and work towards a balance in gut health.

## Food sensitivities

Individuals who struggle with small intestinal bacterial overgrowth (SIBO) may have difficulty digesting certain foods, leading to an array of uncomfortable symptoms. Specifically, high-FODMAP foods, such as onions and garlic, can exacerbate these symptoms, resulting in food sensitivities.

These sensitivities can manifest in various ways, including bloating, gas, abdominal pain, constipation, or diarrhea. In addition to onions and garlic, other high-FODMAP foods commonly linked with SIBO include dairy, wheat, and legumes. Therefore, it is recommended that SIBO sufferers avoid these foods to prevent further discomfort and digestive issues.

If you're experiencing any of these symptoms, it's important to talk to your doctor about getting tested for SIBO. With the right diagnosis and treatment plan, you can alleviate your symptoms and improve your overall quality of life.

## Factors that cause SIBO

There is no exact source for when and where we get SIBO. It can be from the food, drinks, and drugs we intake. Studies show that the factors that may lead to the development of SIBO are the following:

## Low stomach acid

Various factors can cause small intestinal bacterial overgrowth (SIBO), including low stomach acid. This condition can occur due to aging, certain medications, or conditions such as hypochlorhydria and autoimmune gastritis.

SIBO is commonly associated with symptoms such as bloating, gas, and abdominal pain, as well as chronic health issues including autoimmune disease, fibromyalgia, and irritable bowel syndrome. While treatment may include antibiotics and dietary modifications, it is important to address the underlying cause of low stomach acid to prevent the recurrence of SIBO.

## Impaired gut motility

Impaired gut motility, or the inability of the digestive tract muscles to properly move food, can lead to serious health complications such as small intestinal bacterial overgrowth (SIBO). When food remains stagnant in one area for too long, it creates an optimal environment for bacteria to grow and multiply.

This overgrowth of bacteria in the small intestine can lead to symptoms such as abdominal pain, bloating, diarrhea, and malabsorption of nutrients. SIBO has been linked to numerous underlying health conditions, such as hypothyroidism, celiac disease, and diabetes, and can be difficult to diagnose and treat. Maintaining healthy gut motility is crucial for overall digestive health and the prevention of SIBO.

## Structural abnormalities

Factors that cause structural abnormalities in the digestive tract frequently contribute to SIBO. Past surgeries, like those involving the small intestine, or certain conditions, such as Crohn's disease, can interfere with the muscular activity that propels food through the digestive system.

Slowly emptying bowels and weakened digestive muscles can lead to bacterial overgrowth in the small intestine. This overgrowth occurs when gut bacteria migrate upward and colonize the small intestine, compromising the efficacy of the digestive process.

These structural complications can cause symptoms such as bloating, abdominal discomfort, excessive gas, and diarrhea. Hence, identifying and addressing these structural abnormalities is a critical component in the management of SIBO.

## Use of antibiotics

Antibiotic use is just one of many factors that contribute to small intestinal bacterial overgrowth (SIBO). Antibiotics not only wipe out harmful bacteria but also good ones, leading to an imbalance in the gut microbiome.

This imbalance creates conditions that favor the growth and multiplication of harmful bacteria in the small intestine. Additionally, antibiotic use can disrupt the normal motility of the intestines, which further exacerbates the condition. Imbalanced gut flora and compromised gut motility are key factors that contribute to the development of SIBO. Therefore, it's essential to be cautious with antibiotic use and prioritize maintaining a healthy gut microbiome to minimize the risk of SIBO.

## Immune system dysfunction

SIBO, or small intestine bacterial overgrowth, occurs when there is an abnormal increase in the number of bacteria in the small intestine. Immune system dysfunction is just one of many potential causes for this. When the immune system is impaired, harmful bacteria can flourish in the small intestine, leading to symptoms such as bloating, diarrhea, and abdominal pain.

## Dietary factors

Eating a high-carbohydrate or high-sugar diet can feed the bacteria in the gut, leading to overgrowth. SIBO, or small intestinal bacterial overgrowth, can occur when the bacteria in the gut are fed a high-carbohydrate or high-sugar diet.

This overgrowth can lead to uncomfortable symptoms such as bloating, gas, and abdominal pain. Additionally, SIBO can interfere with the proper absorption of nutrients and can potentially cause malnutrition. It is important to maintain a balanced and varied diet to prevent the proliferation of harmful bacteria in the gut.

## Stress

When people experience chronic stress, their bodies release stress hormones that can negatively impact the gut microbiota. Over time, this can lead to imbalances in the microbial ecosystem and, subsequently, SIBO.

To add to this, stress has also been shown to slow down the movement of the gut, resulting in decreased elimination of bacteria and further increasing the risk of SIBO. Therefore, it is important to manage stress levels as part of an overall strategy to prevent this debilitating gastrointestinal ailment.

## Age

SIBO, or small intestinal bacterial overgrowth, is a condition that affects older adults due to factors like changes in gut motility and decreased production of stomach acid. The aging process causes a reduction in gut motility, leading to the stasis of food in the small intestine, thus offering favorable conditions for bacterial growth.

In addition, impaired stomach acid secretion in the elderly can also promote an overgrowth of bacteria. These factors can lead to unpleasant symptoms such as bloating, gas, abdominal pain, diarrhea, and malabsorption of nutrients. Therefore, it is essential to manage the risk factors that cause SIBO in older adults to prevent complications.

If you're experiencing symptoms of SIBO, it's important to speak with a healthcare professional to determine the underlying cause and develop an effective treatment plan. By addressing the root cause of SIBO, you can alleviate your symptoms and improve your overall health.

Researchers found that 80% of IBS patients are positive for SIBO. IBS and SIBO have the same symptoms, but many other factors cause IBS and only one of those factors is SIBO.

## Medical Treatments for SIBO

### Antibiotics

The medical treatment of SIBO often involves antibiotics to eliminate harmful bacteria residing in the gut. Various antibiotics may be used, depending on the severity of the condition.

Rifaximin is reportedly the most effective, with low risks of resistance or side effects. However, some studies indicate that other antibiotics like neomycin and doxycycline can also produce positive results. Importantly, any antibiotic treatment for SIBO needs to be tailored according to an individual's symptoms and goals, as well as previous exposure to antibiotics.

## Probiotics

When it comes to treating small intestinal bacterial overgrowth (SIBO), probiotics have shown efficacy in reducing symptoms like bloating and gas. However, the type of probiotic strain matters. Lactobacillus and Bifidobacterium species are more effective in reducing SIBO symptoms compared to other strains.

Additionally, SIBO patients may need a higher dose of probiotics than those with a healthy gut microbiome. While probiotics can be helpful for SIBO management, it should be noted that they may not be a suitable intervention for all individuals, and consulting with a healthcare professional is recommended.

## Herbal remedies

Small intestinal bacterial overgrowth (SIBO) is a chronic gastrointestinal condition that is notoriously difficult to treat. However, certain herbal remedies have emerged as effective alternatives to traditional antibiotics. Oregano oil, for instance, is particularly effective in reducing the overgrowth of harmful bacteria in the gut.

Garlic is also a potent antimicrobial agent that has been used for centuries to fight off various infections. Similarly, berberine, a compound extracted from plants like goldenseal and barberry, has been found to have strong antimicrobial effects against a range of bacteria, including some of the most drug-resistant strains.

These herbal remedies offer a promising avenue for natural relief from the symptoms of SIBO as well as a potentially safer and more sustainable alternative to conventional antibiotics.

## Elemental diet

An elemental diet, which involves consuming a liquid formula devoid of carbohydrates, is a highly effective option in the management of SIBO. By depriving the harmful bacteria in the gut of carbohydrates, an elemental diet can reduce gut inflammation and promote the healing of the gastrointestinal tract.

However, it is important to consult a medical professional before starting any medical treatment for SIBO to ensure proper diagnosis and management.

## Gut motility agents

Medical treatments for SIBO include gut motility agents, such as prokinetic medications, which can help stimulate the movement of food through the digestive tract. These medications work by increasing the strength and frequency of muscle contractions in the GI tract, allowing food to move more efficiently.

Examples of prokinetic medications used for SIBO include metoclopramide and cisapride. It is important to note that the use of gut motility agents in SIBO should be done under the guidance of a healthcare professional, as their use can have potential side effects and interactions with other medications.

## Diet modifications

In the treatment of SIBO, low-FODMAP diets prove to be effective in reducing the symptoms by decreasing the number of fermentable carbohydrates that feed harmful bacteria. When used in combination with other medical treatments, such as antibiotics, probiotics, and elemental diets, the results are enhanced, and the symptoms of SIBO are further alleviated.

Incorporating these medically prescribed treatments into the low-FODMAP diet can lead to a significant improvement in SIBO symptoms and provide patients with the relief they need to live a more comfortable life.

It's important to note that the best course of treatment for SIBO will vary depending on the individual and the severity of their condition. A healthcare professional can help determine the most appropriate course of treatment to alleviate symptoms and restore gut health.

## Lifestyle Changes of SIBO

Here are some lifestyle changes that can help manage SIBO:

- **Stress reduction:** Stress can hurt gut health, so managing stress is important for individuals with

SIBO. Relaxation techniques like meditation, yoga, and massage can help alleviate stress.

- **Regular exercise:** Exercise can help stimulate gut motility, reducing the risk of bacterial overgrowth. It can also help reduce stress, leading to improved gut health.
- **Sleep hygiene:** Good sleep hygiene, including getting enough rest and establishing a sleep routine, can help reduce stress and improve overall gut health.
- **Hydration:** Drinking plenty of water can help improve gut motility and prevent constipation, reducing the risk of SIBO.
- **Avoid smoking or excess alcohol consumption:** Both smoking and excess alcohol consumption can be detrimental to gut health, potentially leading to SIBO, so avoiding these habits is important.
- **Dealing with underlying conditions:** Certain underlying medical conditions like celiac disease or immune system dysfunction can contribute to SIBO. Treating these conditions can improve gut health overall.
- **Work with a professional:** Individuals with SIBO need to work with a medical professional to develop a personalized treatment plan that includes medical interventions as well as lifestyle changes.

By incorporating these lifestyle changes into their routine, individuals with SIBO can effectively manage their symptoms and improve their overall gut health.

# ALL ABOUT THE SIBO DIET

A SIBO diet can be an effective way to help manage the symptoms of small intestinal bacterial overgrowth (SIBO). If you're living with this condition, it's important to understand how dietary changes can make a big difference in your quality of life.

SIBO is a condition where excessive intestinal bacteria interfere with digestion and the absorption of nutrients, leading to uncomfortable digestive symptoms like gas, bloating, abdominal discomfort, and diarrhea. There are several medical treatments for SIBO as well as lifestyle changes that can help manage its symptoms. One effective approach is the SIBO diet.

## Main principles of a SIBO diet

### Limit fermentable carbohydrates

A SIBO diet focuses on limiting fermentable carbohydrates, which are sugars and complex carbohydrates found in certain fruits, vegetables, grains, and dairy products. Reducing these types of carbs helps to decrease bacterial overgrowth in the small intestine.

Additionally, a SIBO diet typically emphasizes lean protein sources, healthy fats, and non-starchy vegetables. Some recommended foods include salmon, avocado, kale, and green beans. Overall, the goal of a SIBO diet is to eliminate foods that feed bacteria and promote a healthy gut microbiome.

## Avoid processed foods

The main principles of a SIBO diet are to limit or avoid high FODMAP foods, eliminate processed foods that contain additives and preservatives, and consume gut-friendly foods such as fermented vegetables, bone broth, and healthy fats. Incorporating these dietary changes can help alleviate symptoms such as bloating, gas, constipation, and diarrhea. It is important to consult with a healthcare professional before making any significant dietary changes, as each individual's needs may vary.

## Increase dietary fiber

Individuals with SIBO should adhere to a diet high in fiber, as it helps promote healthy digestion and alleviate constipation. Foods such as vegetables, fruits, whole grains, and legumes are excellent sources of dietary fiber. However, it is important to note that some types of fiber, particularly fermentable fibers, may exacerbate symptoms of SIBO.

It is recommended to work with a healthcare provider or registered dietitian to tailor a SIBO diet that is specific to individual needs and symptom management. Additionally, it is essential to avoid foods that are high in sugar, refined carbohydrates, and fiber, as they can exacerbate SIBO symptoms.

### Eat on a regular schedule

To improve gut health, it's important to adhere to certain principles outlined in a SIBO diet. These principles include eating regularly at consistent times throughout the day to maintain digestive processes, limiting or eliminating certain high-FODMAP foods that are known to trigger SIBO symptoms, and incorporating fiber-rich foods to promote healthy gut flora.

It's also important to stay hydrated and minimize stress, as both can adversely affect gut health. Following these principles can help alleviate symptoms and support overall gut health.

### Choose nutrient-dense options

SIBO, a common digestive disorder, disrupts the normal balance of bacteria in the small intestine, leading to uncomfortable symptoms. A nutrient-dense diet is a key factor in managing SIBO by promoting gut health and reducing fermentable carbohydrates that trigger symptoms.

Choosing leafy greens, lean proteins, nuts and seeds, avocados, and fermented vegetables not only provides essential nutrients but also decreases inflammation and promotes a healthier gut microbiome. Those with SIBO need to consult with a qualified healthcare practitioner to develop a personalized plan that addresses their specific needs.

By following these simple principles, individuals with SIBO can reduce their discomfort while also maintaining a balanced diet that provides adequate nourishment.

## Benefits of the SIBO Diet

### Improved Digestion

The SIBO diet offers a range of benefits to those suffering from digestive issues, including the reduction of uncomfortable symptoms like bloating and discomfort. By reducing fermentable carbohydrates and increasing dietary fiber intake, the diet can also improve digestion and aid in the prevention of future flare-ups.

Studies have shown that a low-fermentable oligosaccharides, disaccharides, monosaccharides, and polyols (FODMAP) diet, which is commonly used to manage SIBO, can be effective in reducing symptoms in up to 86% of patients.

Additionally, the SIBO diet can help restore balance to the gut microbiome, further improving digestive health. Overall, incorporating the SIBO diet into one's lifestyle offers a holistic approach to managing and alleviating symptoms related to SIBO.

### Reduced Inflammation

The SIBO diet offers numerous benefits to those suffering from small intestinal bacterial overgrowth (SIBO), including reduced inflammation in the gut by eliminating high-sugar processed foods, which are known to be inflammatory. Besides, it aids in restoring a healthy balance of gut bacteria and alleviates symptoms such as bloating, abdominal pain, and irregular bowel movements.

By adopting this diet, people can improve their overall gut health and experience less discomfort and improved digestion. Additionally, it enables individuals to identify and address any underlying food sensitivities that may be contributing to their symptoms, leading to long-term health benefits.

## Nutrient-Dense Options

The SIBO diet, with its focus on nutrient-dense foods like leafy greens, lean proteins, nuts and seeds, avocados, and fermented vegetables, offers numerous benefits to those suffering from digestive issues. By eliminating complex carbohydrates and added sugars, the diet helps ease symptoms of bloating, gas, and abdominal pain.

Additionally, the diet supplies essential vitamins and minerals that support overall health and well-being. By incorporating these smart food choices, SIBO patients can achieve a balanced, nourishing diet that supports digestive health and optimal nutrition.

## Increased Regularity

One of the key benefits of the SIBO diet is its ability to improve gut health. While developing a regular eating pattern is important, this particular diet goes a step further by targeting small intestinal bacterial overgrowth (SIBO). By eliminating foods that exacerbate SIBO symptoms and incorporating supplements and low-FODMAP foods, individuals may experience reduced bloating, improved nutrient absorption, and better overall gut function.

Additionally, this approach may alleviate other symptoms commonly associated with SIBO, such as gas and discomfort. While further research is needed on this topic, many individuals have reported positive outcomes from following the SIBO diet.

These benefits will help lead to an improved quality of life and allow those with SIBO to manage their condition effectively. By understanding the principles of a SIBO diet, individuals with this condition can find relief from its symptoms and improve their overall gut health.

## Disadvantages of the SIBO Diet

### Restrictive

The SIBO diet, while effective in managing symptoms of small intestinal bacterial overgrowth (SIBO), presents some major disadvantages. Its restrictive nature eliminates a great deal of high-FODMAP foods, such as garlic and onions, making it challenging to follow and potentially limiting food choices.

This can result in nutrient deficiencies and a heightened risk of disordered eating behavior. Furthermore, research shows that adherence to the SIBO diet is difficult and may have limited long-term success in eradicating SIBO.

## Socially Awkward

The SIBO diet can be challenging to maintain, particularly in social settings where the necessary dietary restrictions may not be understood. Those who adhere to the diet must be vigilant about avoiding certain foods and may feel embarrassed or awkward when asking questions or requesting special accommodations at restaurants.

Limitations on diet can also make grocery shopping and meal planning more complicated, requiring careful attention to avoid trigger foods that could cause uncomfortable digestive symptoms. Despite these challenges, many SIBO sufferers find relief from symptoms by making dietary changes, making the inconvenience of the diet worthwhile in the end.

## Requires Patience

One of the main disadvantages of the SIBO diet is that it requires a lot of patience. It can take time, discipline, and persistence to see significant improvements in symptoms. This is not a quick fix or an overnight solution to gut issues. The SIBO diet involves strict adherence to a low-FODMAP diet and the elimination of certain foods that can exacerbate symptoms.

It can take months for the gut to heal and for symptoms to start to improve. The SIBO diet also requires a lot of planning, preparation, and cooking, which can be time-consuming and expensive. However, the potential benefits of the SIBO diet are significant, as it can lead to improved gut health, reduced inflammation, and relief from symptoms.

Although the disadvantages of the SIBO diet may occur, the benefits will far outweigh the disadvantages in the long run. With a proper understanding of the SIBO diet and its principles, individuals with this condition can find relief from its symptoms and improve their quality of life.

By following these simple guidelines, those with SIBO can reduce their uncomfortable digestive symptoms while still maintaining a balanced diet that provides adequate nourishment.

# GETTING STARTED WITH THE SIBO DIET

Before you begin the diet, you should assess your current eating habits and identify any high-FODMAP foods that need to be eliminated. Once you have recognized these items, you can create a diet plan that works for you and your lifestyle.

**5-Step Guide on Getting Started the SIBO Diet**

The SIBO diet is a specialized approach to managing digestive issues caused by small intestinal bacterial overgrowth. If you're considering this diet, it's important to follow the proper steps for success.

- **Step 1: Consult your doctor**

Ask your doctor or registered dietitian to ensure that the SIBO diet is appropriate for your individual needs. This professional can also help tailor the plan to meet your specific dietary requirements and provide guidance on supplementation. With their support, you can get started with confidence and improve your gut health.

- **Step 2: Eliminate high-FODMAP foods**

The second step is particularly crucial as it entails eliminating high-FODMAP foods known to cause gut inflammation and exacerbate SIBO symptoms. Lactose, fructose, and polyols are among the high-FODMAP foods to be avoided. Despite the daunting nature of this step, numerous resources are available to guide one through the process.

These include dieticians, meal plans, and online resources geared towards the elimination of high-FODMAP foods. By following this step, individuals with SIBO can manage their symptoms and promote long-term gut health.

- **Step 3: Focus on low-starch vegetables**

As per the Main 5-Step Guide on Getting Started with the SIBO Diet, Step 3 involves focusing on low-starchy vegetables that are rich in essential vitamins and minerals and low in fermentable fibers. These vegetables, such as broccoli, cauliflower, kale, and spinach, help in starving off the excessive bacterial growth in the gut, thus promoting a healthy gut environment.

They are also easily digested, making them a perfect addition to a SIBO-friendly diet. Additionally, the low-starch content of these vegetables helps in reducing inflammation and promoting overall gut health. So, if you're looking to start a SIBO diet, make sure to add these low-starchy vegetables to your grocery list.

- **Step 4: Incorporate healthy fats**

Incorporating healthy fats is a crucial step in the SIBO diet, which aims to alleviate the symptoms of small intestinal bacterial overgrowth. The diet's main goal is to reduce the growth of bacteria in the small intestines by eliminating foods that feed the bacteria.

Healthy fats, such as olive oil, coconut oil, and avocado, improve nutrient absorption and help reduce inflammation in the body. Furthermore, consuming healthy fats does not worsen SIBO symptoms, as they are easily digestible and do not trigger bacterial overgrowth. Thus, adding these oils to the SIBO diet can have a positive impact on overall health and well-being.

- **Step 5: Introduce probiotics and prebiotics**

In step five of the SIBO diet, incorporating probiotics and prebiotics can have a significant impact on gut health. Probiotic supplements work to replenish and maintain the good bacteria in the gut, while prebiotics provide the necessary fuel for these bacteria to flourish.

However, it is important to consult with a healthcare professional before adding these supplements to the diet. The SIBO diet's 5-Step Guide stresses the significance of taking a personalized approach to the diet and supplement regimen and seeking guidance from a qualified healthcare practitioner.

By following these steps, you'll be well on your way to starting the SIBO diet and promoting gut health. Just remember to be patient, take it one step at a time, and seek guidance from a healthcare professional if needed.

## Foods to eat

Here are some examples of foods to eat while following the SIBO diet:

- **Low FODMAP Fruits:** Fruits that are low in FODMAPs, such as unripe bananas, strawberries, and cantaloupe, can be enjoyed in moderation. These fruits provide vitamins and antioxidants without triggering gut inflammation or exacerbating SIBO symptoms. Plus, they make a great snack!
- **Low-Starch Vegetables:** When following the SIBO diet, it's important to focus on low-starch vegetables like green beans, cucumbers, and spinach. These vegetables are low in fermentable fibers and easy to digest, making them a safe option for those with SIBO. Plus, they add color and nutrition to any meal!
- **Healthy Proteins:** Healthy proteins such as grass-fed beef, wild-caught fish, and organic poultry provide essential amino acids for building and repairing tissues. It's important to choose high-quality, grass-fed, or wild-caught meats and avoid processed options that often contain added sugars, fillers, and preservatives. Plus, protein is essential for satiety and muscle growth!
- **Healthy Fats:** Healthy fats such as olive oil, coconut oil, and avocado provide essential fatty acids that help reduce inflammation and improve overall health. These healthy fats also help keep you fuller for longer and can help regulate blood sugar levels. Plus, they add flavor and richness to any dish!

- **Herbs and Spices:** Herbs and spices such as ginger, turmeric, and oregano offer a host of health benefits and can be used to add flavor to SIBO-friendly meals. In addition to their anti-inflammatory properties, many herbs and spices also have antibacterial properties that can help fight off SIBO. Plus, they add variety and depth of flavor to any dish!

By incorporating these foods into their diet, those with SIBO can promote gut health and reduce inflammation. As always, it's important to listen to your body and make adjustments to your diet as needed. Plus, with so many delicious options available, there's no reason not to enjoy the SIBO diet!

**Foods to avoid**

Here are some examples of foods to avoid while following the SIBO diet:

- **High FODMAP Fruits:** Fruits that are high in FODMAPs, such as apples, peaches, and mangoes, should be avoided while following the SIBO diet. These fruits are high in fermentable fibers and can trigger gut inflammation and exacerbate SIBO symptoms.
- **High-Starch Vegetables:** High-starch vegetables like potatoes and sweet potatoes should be avoided while following the SIBO diet. These vegetables are difficult to digest and can exacerbate gut inflammation, leading to uncomfortable symptoms.

- **Processed Foods:** Processed foods that are high in sugar, additives, and preservatives can exacerbate symptoms of SIBO. These foods can also cause inflammation throughout the body and may lead to the overgrowth of harmful bacteria in the gut.

- **Gluten-Containing Grains:** Grains such as wheat, barley, and rye contain gluten, which can exacerbate symptoms of gut inflammation and SIBO. It's essential to avoid these grains and instead opt for gluten-free alternatives like quinoa, rice, and oats.

- **Dairy Products:** Dairy products like milk, cheese, and yogurt contain lactose, which can exacerbate symptoms of gut inflammation and SIBO.Those with lactose intolerance or SIBO should avoid dairy products or opt for lactose-free alternatives.

By avoiding these foods while following the SIBO diet, those with SIBO can reduce inflammation, promote gut health, and alleviate uncomfortable symptoms. As always, it's important to listen to your body and make adjustments to your diet as needed.

# WEEK 1: LIMITING OF FOOD WITH FODMAPS

This chapter starts the weekly tasks to reverse the symptoms of SIBO. The first thing to do when you have SIBO is to limit yourself to eating foods containing FODMAPs. This task should be done for 6 to 8 weeks. The major components of FODMAPs are explained in detail here and the specific foods needed to be avoided or limited and the foods you are allowed to eat are listed.

## FODMAPs Major Components

FODMAP foods contain the following major carbs that are hard to digest. Below are their definitions and the food allowed to avoid so FODMAPs consumption is lowered.

### Lactose

Lactose is a sugar molecule found in cow's, sheep's, and goat's milk. It is a carbohydrate from dairy products. People with Lactose intolerance do not have or lack the enzyme lactase that digests lactose. Lactose that is not digested properly causes abdominal bloating, gas, pain, and diarrhea. The effect usually occurs 30 minutes up to hours after the consumption of dairy products.

**Avoid foods such as:**

- Cow's, Sheep's, and Goat's milk
- Ice cream with milk
- Yogurts from Cow and Soy Yogurt
- Whipping Cream
- Soy milk
- Cottage, Ricotta and Mascarpone Cheese
- Sour Cream

**Food allowed:**

- Milk from almond, coconut, hazelnut, hemp, and rice
- Cream Cheese
- Coconut milk yogurt
- Butter
- Hard cheeses such as Swiss, cheddar, blue cheese, brie, parmesan, mozzarella, and feta

**Fructose**

Fructose is the simple sugar found in fruits, high-fructose corn syrup (HFCS), honey, vegetables, and agave syrup. The lack of enzymes that digest fructose is called Fructose Malabsorption. The absorption of fructose depends on another sugar or carbohydrate called glucose. Foods containing fructose and glucose with a 1:1 ratio are tolerated by a person with SIBO but once the ratio changes the food is to be avoided.

**Food to avoid:**

**Fruits**

- Apricots
- Apples
- Nectarines
- Pears
- Raspberries
- Blackberries
- Cherries
- Watermelon
- White Peaches
- Papaya
- Plums
- Peaches
- Canned Fruit
- Prunes
- Mango
- Persimmon
- Large portions of any fruit
- Orange

**Vegetables**

- Pumpkin
- Artichokes
- Asparagus
- Garlic
- Onions

- Green peppers
- Shallot
- Leek
- Cabbage
- Cauliflower
- Sugar snap peas
- Mushrooms

**Food to consume:**

**Fruits**

- Lime
- Banana
- Strawberries
- Tangelos
- Cantaloupe
- Pineapple
- Honeydew
- Blueberries
- Grapefruit
- Lemon
- Sugar snap peas
- Grapes
- Kiwi
- Rhubarb

**Vegetables**

- Red bell pepper
- Lettuce
- Green Beans
- Spinach
- Bean sprouts
- Cucumber
- Carrots
- Chives
- Eggplant
- Tomato
- Bok choy
- Water Chestnuts
- Potatoes

## Fructan

When the intestine lacks an enzyme to break the fructose-to-fructose bond, some carbohydrates are completely malabsorbed, and they are called Fructans. Fructans also cause gas, bloating, and pain. The majority of a person's fructan intake is from wheat.

**Food to avoid:**

- Spelt
- Wheat
- Rye
- Barley

**Food to consume:**

- Corn
- Brown Rice
- Quinoa
- Oats, Oat Bran
- Gluten-free bread, cereals, pasta, crackers, apple/pear juice, agave or HFCS
- Namaste Food Perfect Flour Blend or King Arthur Gluten Free
- Multi-Purpose Flour

## Galactans

When a person lacks enzymes to digest the fructose-to-fructose bond, aside from fructan, a carbohydrate called Galactan is also produced. It was usually caused by the consumption of beans and lentils.

**Food to avoid:**

- Baked Beans
- Kidney Beans
- Hummus
- Edamame
- Lentils
- Chickpeas
- Soy milk
- Pistachios

**Food to consume:**

- Peanuts
- Less than 1/3 cup of green peas
- Tofu
- One to two tablespoons of almonds, macadamia, pecans, pine nuts, walnuts, pumpkin seed, sesame seed, sunflower seed

## Polyols

Polyols are also called sugar alcohols. They are often used as sweeteners. Naturally, Polyols are found in fruits and vegetables and are usually the sweeteners for mints, cough drops, sugar-free gums, and medications.

**Food to avoid:**

- Honey
- Inulin
- High fructose corn syrup
- Splenda
- Rum
- Agave
- Sorbitol, Mannitol, Xylitol, Maltitol
- Sugar alcohols (sweeteners)
- Chicory root
- Fructose-oligosaccharides (FOS)

**Food to consume:**

- Canola oil
- Pure maple syrup

- Sugar
- Glucose, sucrose
- Aspartame
- Vodka, gin (limited to one serving)
- Fish
- Eggs
- Olives
- Meat
- Chicken
- Turkey
- Wine, beer

Limiting FODMAPs will probably be a major change in your usual diet but you have helped yourself recover from SIBO. Chapter 7 provides different recipes for meals that you can try to make for your SIBO diet.

# WEEK 2: FASTING

Lapine (2018) suggests that the SIBO diet is not only by which food you are allowed to eat but also by the manner you eat the food. The manner you eat might as well be the prime reason you have SIBO anyway. Aside from the food to eat and avoid, SIBO can also be minimized through fasting. These lifestyles can help normalize stomach movement and bacteria better than the diet itself.

## The Intermittent Fasting

Intermittent fasting is a dieting method that works by alternating periods of calorie restriction with eating windows. When it comes to managing SIBO, intermittent fasting can be helpful by limiting the amount of food available for bacteria in the small intestine to feed on. This reduction in bacterial activity adds an extra line of defense against SIBO by maintaining the much-needed sterility of the small intestine.

To begin, individuals should consider starting with a 12 to 14-hour overnight fast and gradually working their way up until they reach an optimal fasting period of 16 to 24 hours. During fasting hours, the body relies on internal sources for energy and may even use stored fat cells for energy. During eating windows, it's essential to consume a nutrient-dense meal to provide the body with the vital vitamins and minerals necessary for healthy gut function.

Intermittent fasting can also help reduce overall inflammation, which is a prevailing issue associated with SIBO. By regulating insulin sensitivity and promoting autophagy, the body may be able to better reduce inflammation and repair tissues damaged by SIBO.

It's crucial to remember that intermittent fasting is not for everyone and should always be done with the guidance of a healthcare professional. Those with certain medical conditions and pregnant or breastfeeding individuals should not attempt intermittent fasting without discussing it with their doctor.

Overall, intermittent fasting can be a useful tool in managing SIBO by limiting bacterial growth and maintaining healthy gut function, but it's essential to ensure that it's the right dietary approach for each individual before beginning.

# WEEK 3: SIBO BEVERAGES

Welcome to week 3 of the SIBO diet! During this week, it's important to continue following the low-FODMAP, low-starch, and anti-inflammatory diet plan while also incorporating SIBO-friendly beverages. Keeping hydrated is essential for gut health and can help alleviate symptoms of SIBO.

Many beverages are rich in probiotics and nutrients that promote gut healing and reduce inflammation. This week, the focus is on choosing beverages that are hydrating, nutritious, and gut-healing.

From herbal teas to coconut water, there's no shortage of delicious and healthy beverage options for those with SIBO. Let's dive in and explore some of the best SIBO-friendly beverages to enjoy during Week 3 of the SIBO diet!

- **Water:** Staying hydrated is essential for gut health, and water is always a great choice for those with SIBO.Drinking plenty of water can add to feelings of fullness and aid in the digestion of food.
- **Herbal Teas:** Herbal teas like peppermint, ginger, and chamomile are excellent choices for those with SIBO. These teas have anti-inflammatory and anti-

bacterial properties that can help soothe the gut and alleviate uncomfortable symptoms.

- **Coconut Water:** Coconut water is a naturally hydrating and nutrient-rich beverage that can help replenish electrolytes and promote gut health. It's important to choose coconut water that is free from added sugars or additives.

- **Bone Broth:** Bone broth is a nutrient-dense and gut-healing beverage that is easy to digest and can help promote healthy digestion. It's important to choose bone broth that is made from high-quality, grass-fed, or organic animal bones.

- **Kombucha:** Kombucha is a fermented beverage made from tea and sugar that contains beneficial probiotics for gut health. It's important to choose kombucha that is low in sugar and free from added flavors or additives.

By incorporating these SIBO-friendly beverages into their diets those with SIBO can promote gut health and reduce inflammation. Plus, with so many delicious options available, staying hydrated has never been so tasty!

This task should be done simultaneously with all the other weekly tasks. You can also continue doing this even after the symptoms are reversed because this task gives our stomach a lot of benefits.

# WEEK 4: DIETARY SUPPLEMENTS

Week 4 of the SIBO diet calls for incorporating dietary supplements that can help manage symptoms and promote gut health. From probiotics to herbal teas, there is a wide range of supplements available that can provide relief from symptoms such as bloating and gas and help reduce inflammation in the gut.

- **Probiotics:** Probiotics are beneficial bacteria that help support a healthy gut microbiome. Taking probiotic supplements can help replenish good bacteria in the digestive tract and promote gut health.

- **Digestive Enzymes:** Digestive enzymes can help break down food and aid in digestion. Taking digestive enzyme supplements is a great way to reduce symptoms of bloating and gas.

- **Herbal Supplements:** Herbal supplements like turmeric, ginger, licorice root, and oregano oil have anti-inflammatory properties that can help reduce inflammation in the gut. These herbal supplements may also help regulate levels of good and bad bacteria in the digestive tract.

More supplements can help reverse the symptoms of SIBO. Remember, when taking a supplement, the only goal is to kill the bad bacteria by not feeding or washing them away. Also, supplements add good bacteria and helpful acids to our stomachs.

# WEEK 5: REINTRODUCTION OF FOOD

Notice that we skip weeks 5 and 6, and we jump right straight into week 7. You should continue limiting your intake of foods with FODMAPs for a minimum of 6 weeks. You can discontinue fasting or dietary supplements, but of course, the more you do to ease the SIBO symptoms, the more you will feel better. Also, nutritionists recommend starting this task usually in the 7th week.

## Reintroduction of food

Week 7 is a crucial phase in the SIBO diet as it involves the reintroduction of certain foods into the diet to see how well they're tolerated. During this week, individuals should focus on one particular food group, such as dairy or grains, to test their tolerance levels to these foods.

If the person tolerates the food group without any adverse symptoms, they can gradually add more variety over the week and monitor any reactions.

It's essential to take note of any symptoms that might arise during the reintroduction period, such as bloating, gas, or constipation, as they can provide clues as to which foods are best avoided.

The reintroduction period should be done slowly, with only one new food introduced at a time to ensure it's easy to pinpoint which food might be causing a reaction. It's also important to ensure that the foods being reintroduced are of high quality and free from common additives and preservatives that may irritate the gut.

Individuals should continue to follow the SIBO diet during the reintroduction phase to ensure that no new bacterial overgrowth occurs due to compromised gut function. Once the reintroduction phase is complete, individuals may work with a registered dietitian to establish a long-term diet plan that fits their unique nutritional needs and digestive health requirements.

### Sample Meal Plan and  Selected Recipes

Here is a sample meal plan made for a week that you can either follow or modify accordingly. The meals listed below are lifted from the sample recipes included in this guide. The purpose of creating a meal plan is to help you to watch what you are about to consume and make sure you're meeting your daily nutrition needs.

|  | AM<br>(breakfast and snack) | Noon<br>(lunch and snack) | PM<br>(dinner) |
|---|---|---|---|
| **Day 1** | Celery root hash browns with sauteed spinach<br>Scrambled eggs | Tuna salad with arugula and cucumber | Roasted cabbage<br>Roasted salmon with a side of green beans |
|  | Carrot cake muffins | Bone broth |  |
| **Day 2** | Pumpkin pie with coconut cream<br>A side of berries | Asian bowl medley with ginger chicken<br>Shredded carrots | Shepherd's pie with ground beef<br>Mashed sweet potatoes broccoli |
|  | Baked salmon with lemon juice | Bone broth |  |
| **Day 3** | Greek yogurt with sliced peaches<br>Chopped almonds | Mexican steak salad with mixed greens<br>Avocado | Baked salmon with blueberry sauce<br>A side of roasted Brussels sprouts |
|  | Carrot cake muffins | Bone broth |  |
| **Day 4** | Scrambled eggs with spinach<br>Roasted sweet potatoes | Roasted cabbage<br>Ginger chicken salad | Grilled salmon with asparagus<br>Cauliflower rice |
|  | Carrot sticks with almond butter | Coconut yogurt with blueberries |  |

|  | AM<br>(breakfast and snack) | Noon<br>(lunch and snack) | PM<br>(dinner) |
|---|---|---|---|
| **Day 5** | Coconut flour pancakes with berries and coconut cream | Tuna salad with mixed greens<br>Lemon ginger dressing | Shepherd's pie with ground beef<br>Butternut squash |
|  | Bone broth | Carrot cake muffins |  |
| **Day 6** | Smoothie with banana, spinach, almond milk, and collagen protein powder | Mexican steak salad with mixed greens and avocado | Lemon ginger chicken with roasted carrots and parsnips |
|  | Carrot sticks with hummus | Bone broth |  |
| **Day 7** | Almond butter<br>Blueberry smoothie | Asian bowl medley with salmon and sautéed bok choy | Baked salmon with roasted asparagus and mixed greens |
|  | Carrot cake muffins | Bone broth |  |

Remember, this meal plan is intended to be a guide to help you get started on the SIBO diet. Be sure to work with your healthcare provider to customize the plan according to your individual needs and preferences.

Don't forget to listen to your body and adjust accordingly. With the right approach and mindset, you can successfully manage SIBO and enjoy delicious and nutritious meals.

# TOP RECIPES

## Asian Bowl Medley

**Ingredients:**

- 1 tbsp. tomato paste
- 1 red capsicum, diced
- 1 carrot, julienned
- 1 tbsp. lard
- 1 tsp. grated turmeric
- 1 tsp. apple cider vinegar
- 400g free-range pork mince
- 1 zucchini, spirals
- 2 tbsp. coconut aminos
- 4 spring onions, green part only, sliced
- 1 tsp. grated ginger

**Instructions:**

1. Heat over the pan until it is smoking hot.
2. Put in the lard and let it melt. Then add the pork mince and stir occasionally until the pork is cooked through and any liquid is absorbed.

3. Put in the ginger and turmeric and for 1 minute, stir fry the ingredients.
4. Add one vegetable after every 30 seconds, and continue stirring the ingredients during the 30-second interval.
5. Put in a minimal amount of water whenever the wok is getting too dry.
6. Pour in the tomato paste, coconut amino, and apple cider vinegar.
7. Add some salt and pepper as needed.
8. Turn off the heat and serve.

## Mexican Steak Salad

**Ingredients:**

**For the salad:**

- 6 chopped radishes
- bell pepper (red, green, yellow – one of each, chopped)
- 1 tsp. coriander
- 2 medium, heirloom tomatoes
- 1 can hatch green chilies
- 1/2 cabbage- chopped
- 1/2 tsp. black pepper
- 1 can of sliced black olives
- 1 tsp. cumin
- 1 bunch of cilantro

**For the dressing:**

- 1/2 tsp. salt
- 2 tbsp. garlic-infused sesame oil
- 1 freshly squeezed lemon

**For the steak and marinade:**

- 1.5 lbs. of flank steak
- 1 jalapeno, seeds removed
- 1 lb. carrot
- 1/3 cup coconut aminos
- 1 cup coconut vinegar
- 2 tsp. Chipotle powder
- 1 tsp. honey
- 1/2 tsp. salt

**Instructions:**

1. Put all ingredients for the steak marinade into the blender. Pulse until you get a smooth consistency.
2. Pour marinade into a bowl and add steak, let it sit for about one hour.
3. During the one-hour marinating of steak, chop off all the salad ingredients and place them in a bowl.
4. After marinating, cut the steak so it can fit into the skillet. Heat the skillet.
5. Cover the whole pan with sesame oil.
6. Fry both sides of the steak until it is cooked based on your liking.
7. When cooked, let it cool before cutting it into strips.
8. Add beef strips on top of the salad.
9. Add dressing before serving.

# Shepherd's Pie

**Ingredients:**

**For the crust:**

- 2 tbsp. garlic-infused oil
- 1 cup Brazil nuts
- 1/2 tsp. salt
- 1/3 cup palm shortening
- 1/3 cup almond flour

**For the filling:**

- 1 cup frozen peas
- 3/4 lbs. ground turkey thighs
- 1/4 tsp. marjoram
- 1/4 tsp. red pepper flakes
- 1 large carrot
- 2 tbsp. garlic-infused oil
- 1 tsp. salt
- 1/4 tsp. black pepper

**For the topping:**

- 1/4 cup 24 hr. or lactose-free yogurt or you can use dairy-free yogurt, water, or almond milk instead
- 1 Kabocha squash
- 1/2 tsp. salt

## Instructions:

1. Place the Brazil nuts into a food processor and mix until the nuts become a fine powder.
2. Add all the ingredients of the pie crust into a bowl and mix them with your hands so that the oil is pressed.
3. Make a big patty from dough formed from the mixed crust ingredients.
4. Wrap it in parchment paper then place it in the freezer for 30 minutes.
5. Slice the Kabocha squash into 8 fractions and add it to the double boiler.
6. Boil the Kabocha squash until it is soft enough and the meat inside can be easily scooped out. Then put it aside to cool.
7. Put garlic oil in a medium-high heated skillet.
8. Put in salute and carrots until they are brownish.
9. Add in the peas and cook for a few more minutes.
10. Put the vegetables on the side of the skillet and cook the ground turkey in the middle.
11. Add salt and spices as necessary.
12. Press and stir the ground turkey thoroughly so it will not turn into big chunks of meat.
13. When the turkey turns brown, mix it with all the vegetables and sauté until all the ingredients are cooked.
14. Turn off the stove and put the dish aside.
15. Heat the oven to 400 degrees before putting the dough.
16. Put the dough in the baking dish or pie tin and spread it evenly to shape up the crust.
17. Bake the crust for 20 minutes.
18. Remove the seeds of the squash.

19. Peel off the skin of the squash and put it in the Cuisinart together with yogurt and salt. (Instead of yogurt, coconut milk, or almond milk, Water can also be used).
20. Blend the ingredients until it has a smooth texture.
21. After the crust is baked, put the turkey and veggie sauté on the crust.
22. Put the mashed squash on top of the sauté.
23. Bake the pie for 20 minutes.
24. Remove the pie from the oven and let it cool, then serve.

## Carrot Muffin

### Ingredients:

- 2 1/2 tsp cinnamon
- 1 tsp vanilla
- 1/4 cup coconut flour
- 1/4 tsp sea salt
- 1/2 tsp baking soda
- 2 cups shredded carrots
- 3 large eggs
- 1/4 cup coconut oil
- 1/4 cup honey

### Instructions:

1. Preheat the oven to 375°F.
2. Mix the coconut oil, eggs, honey, and vanilla until they produce a smooth texture.

3. In a separate bowl, mix all the dry ingredients. Add the combined dry ingredients to the wet ingredients and gently mix until a batter is formed.
4. Put the shredded carrots and mix until it is incorporated.
5. Put the thick batter into a muffin tray.
6. Place the tray in the oven and bake for 20-25 minutes or until the muffins are springy to the touch or until lightly browned and a toothpick comes out clean.
7. Serve while warm.

## Beef Bone Broth

## Ingredients:

- 2 tbsp. coconut oil or ghee
- sea salt
- 1/2 cup apple cider vinegar
- 2 lbs. beef stew meat
- 3 lbs. beef bone marrow
- 2 tsp. dried thyme or several sprigs of fresh thyme tied together
- 3 carrots, coarsely chopped
- 1 bunch of green onions, green parts only, coarsely chopped
- 1 bunch of parsley
- about 4 or more quarts of cold water
- 3 celery stalks, chop coarsely
- optional: 1 tsp. green peppercorns, dried and crushed, or substitute with freshly ground pepper

## Instructions:

1. Put the bone marrow in a large soup pot together with vinegar and water. Let it stand for about an hour.
2. Heat the oil in a huge frying pan. Put in the stew meat and fry until it turns brown.
3. Transfer the meat and fat you fry from the pan to the pot for soup and add the vegetables.
4. Put some water until it covers the bones and don't let it overflow or become full.
5. Let it boil.
6. Using a wooden spoon, remove any scum that comes to the top.
7. Decrease the heat and add on the crushed peppercorns or ground pepper or thyme.
8. Boil the stock for a minimum of 12 and a maximum of 72 hours.
9. Put water in to maintain the level of water in the beginning.
10. Put in the parsley and let it simmer for 10 minutes more.
11. Using a slotted spoon, remove the stew meat and the bones from the pot. 12. Strain the meat stock and put it into a large bowl and let it cool in the refrigerator.
12. When cooled, remove the fat that will rise at the top.
13. Put into containers and refrigerate.
14. The refrigerated broth should be consumed for up to three days.

# Lemon Ginger Chicken

## Ingredients:

- 1 tbsp. honey
- 6 chicken thighs
- 1 tsp. butter
- 1/2 tsp. coriander
- 1 tbsp. olive oil
- 2 tbsp. ginger, minced
- 1/3 cup wine, white or prosecco, or chicken broth
- 1-1/2 cups carrots, diced
- 2 zucchini, sliced
- 1/2 large lemon, for juice and zest

## Instructions:

1. Fry chicken in butter and olive oil in a pan placed over medium heat until brown.
2. Deglaze the pan with broth or wine and stir to remove the bits on the pan.
3. Add coriander, ginger, and lemon zest to the pan. Cook until half the liquid has evaporated.
4. Remove the chicken.
5. Put the carrots, honey, and lemon juice into the pan.
6. As the carrots start to soften, put back the chicken into the pan, followed by the zucchini.
7. Turn to low and simmer. Add water if needed.
8. To check doneness, pierce the chicken to check if the juice runs clear.
9. Make sure also that the zucchini are tender.

10. If desired, sprinkle with parsley upon serving.

## Salmon with Blueberry Sauce

### Ingredients:

- 1 salmon filet, roughly 1/2" thick
- salt
- 2 tsp. coconut oil
- 1/2 cup blueberries
- 1/2 orange, for juice and zest
- white pepper
- SIBO-friendly blueberry sauce
- 1/4 tsp. freshly grated nutmeg

### Instructions:

1. Mix all the sauce ingredients in a pan on medium-low heat. Stir constantly while cooking the salmon.
2. Once the sauce thickens and the blueberry melts, turn off the stove. Continue cooking the salmon until it's done.
3. Fry the salmon filet with coconut oil. Cook the salmon until it has a light golden color.
4. You can add simple butter-sautéed green beans but remember that the SIBO diet only allows no more than 10 bean pods per serving.
5. A pinch of Hawaiian black lava salt adds a fun flavor.
6. After cooking the salmon, place it next to the green beans then top it with the blueberry sauce and serve.

# Tuna Salad

## Ingredients:

- 1 can tuna, white albacore in spring water
- 2 celery stalks, diced
- 1/2 English cucumber, diced
- 1 Roma tomato, diced
- 2-3 fresh dill sprigs, minced
- 1 small carrot, shredded
- 1/2 large lemon for juice or more to taste
- butter lettuce leaves, torn
- a handful of parsley, fresh Italian or flat-leaf, chopped

## Instructions

1. Start by combining one can of drained albacore tuna in a medium-sized bowl.
2. Add tomato, cucumber, celery, and carrot.
3. Mix in a big handful of parsley and dill.
4. Add the squeezed lemon juice into the mixture and stir until combined.
5. Season to taste with salt, pepper, and garlic powder if desired.
6. Serve over butter lettuce leaves for a delicious, healthy meal!

## Baked Salmon with Ghee

## Ingredients:

- 4 tbsp. ghee or grass-fed butter
- 1–2 lb. wild Alaskan salmon filets
- fresh or dried thyme
- 1 lemon, divided into two

## Instructions:

1. Preheat the oven to 350°F.
2. Spread butter on a baking tray and arrange the salmon filets. Season with salt and pepper.
3. Get half of the lemon and slice thinly. Set aside the other half for baking.
4. Arrange lemon slices on top of the filets. Spread butter over each filet.
5. Add thyme on top of the lemon.
6. Bake the salmon at 350°F for about 10-20 minutes.
7. Duration will depend on how thick or thin the slices are.
8. Squeeze the other half of the lemon on top of the filet before serving.

## Pumpkin Pie

## Ingredients:

- 3 large eggs
- 1-1/2 cups roasted pumpkin puree or canned pumpkin puree
- 1 Paleo Pie Crust, unbaked
- 1/2 cup full-fat coconut milk
- 1/2 cup honey or maple syrup
- 1/8 tsp. Celtic sea salt

- 1 tbsp. pumpkin pie spice

## Instructions:

1. Using a food processor, mix the eggs and pumpkin puree.
2. Add in honey, coconut milk, salt, and pumpkin pie spice.
3. Put the filling into the Paleo Pie Crust
4. Bake for 45 minutes at 350°F.
5. Let it cool then place it in the fridge for 2 hours for it to set up.

## Celery Root Hash Browns

## Ingredients:

- 4 tbsp. tallow butter, or coconut oil
- 2-3 medium celery roots
- 1/2 tsp. sea salt

## Instructions:

1. Using a vegetable peeler or paring knife, scrub and peel the celery root.
2. Grate the root using a cheese grater.
3. Heat a skillet over medium heat and melt tallow in it.
4. When the tallow is already melted, put the grated celery root in the skillet and add salt as necessary.
5. Cook until the ingredients get soft, it usually takes 10 minutes.

6. Turn the heat down and continue to sauté until the hash browns turn brown on the bottom which usually takes another 10 minutes.
7. Flip and cook the other side then serve!

## Roasted Cabbage

### Ingredients:

- 1 tbsp. pepper
- 1 head of cabbage, cut into half- or 1/4-inch
- 1 tbsp. salt
- 3 tbsp.  coconut oil
- 1 tsp. favorite herbs such as basil caraway seeds, and dill (optional)

### Instructions:

1. Preheat the oven to 400°F.
2. Spread a tablespoon of oil on a baking sheet.
3. Put the cabbage on the baking sheet and shower it with the remaining oil.
4. Add salt, pepper, and other spices as necessary. Place it in the oven.
5. Put it in the oven for 35-40 minutes or roast until tender or until the middle and sides start to turn golden brown.
6. Remove it then serve.

# Conclusion

Congratulations! You have made it to the end of this comprehensive guide on SIBO and the SIBO diet. By now, you should have a good understanding of what SIBO is, how it develops, the common symptoms, and the dietary approach to managing it.

It's important to remember that SIBO is a treatable condition, and with proper diagnosis and management, you can regain your quality of life. The SIBO diet, although challenging to follow, has been proven effective in reducing symptoms and preventing relapse.

One of the most critical aspects of managing SIBO is following the SIBO diet as recommended by your healthcare provider. This usually involves reducing your intake of fermentable carbohydrates, including sugars and fibers, which can feed the bacteria in your small intestine.

It's crucial to emphasize that the SIBO diet is not a one-size-fits-all approach, and it may take some time to find the right balance of foods to manage your symptoms effectively. So don't be discouraged if you don't see immediate improvement, but continue to work with your healthcare provider to fine-tune your diet.

In addition to dietary modifications, other lifestyle changes, such as stress management, exercise, and getting enough sleep, can also have a positive impact on managing SIBO symptoms. This is because stress can negatively impact gut motility, which can worsen SIBO, while exercise can help improve it.

With the right combination of diet and lifestyle changes, many people with SIBO can experience significant improvement in their symptoms, allowing them to resume their daily activities without discomfort or embarrassment.

Although SIBO can be a frustrating and isolating condition, it's important to remember that you're not alone. Many others like you are dealing with SIBO symptoms and working towards managing them successfully.

So be kind to yourself as you navigate this journey, and know that it's okay to ask for help and support from your healthcare provider, friends, and family. You may also find it helpful to join a support group or online community of people who understand what you're going through.

In conclusion, managing SIBO requires a multifaceted approach involving a combination of dietary modifications, lifestyle changes, and ongoing support from healthcare providers, family, and friends. Although it can be challenging, with persistence and patience, you can find a way to manage your symptoms and regain your quality of life. So don't give up hope, and remember to celebrate every small victory along the way. Best of luck to you on your journey toward better health and wellness!

# References and Helpful Links

Chris Kresser, M. S. (2022, September 22). What is SIBO? causes, symptoms and treatment. Chris Kresser. Retrieved April 29, 2023, from https://chriskresser.com/sibo-what-causes-it-and-why-its-so-hard-to-treat/.

Diet for IBS and SIBO. (n.d.-a). Retrieved April 29, 2023, from https://www.gidoctor.net/contents/diet-for-ibs-and-sibo.

Diet for those with symptomatic small bowel bacterial overgrowth. (n.d.). Retrieved April 29, 2023, from https://med.virginia.edu/ginutrition/wp-content/uploads/sites/199/2014/04/SBBO-Diet-10-27-16.pdf.

Diet. (n.d.). SIBO - Small Intestinal Bacterial Overgrowth. Retrieved April 29, 2023, from https://www.siboinfo.com/diet.html.

Fodmap food list. (n.d.). IBS Diets. Retrieved April 29, 2023, from https://www.ibsdiets.org/fodmap-diet/fodmap-food-list/.

Lapine, P. (2018, April 4). The best SIBO diets and lifestyle changes for preventing relapse. Feed Me Phoebe. https://feedmephoebe.com/sibo-diet-and-lifestyle-changes/.

Magge, S., & Lembo, A. (2012). Low-fodmap diet for treatment of irritable bowel syndrome. Gastroenterology & Hepatology, 8(11), 739–745. https://www.ncbi.nlm.nih.gov/pmc/articles/PMC3966170/.

SIBO diet: Beneficial foods and foods to avoid. (2018, August 16). Healthline. https://www.healthline.com/health/sibo-diet.

Small intestinal bacterial overgrowth: Updates and clinical implications. (n.d.). Retrieved April 29, 2023, from https://www.youtube.com/watch?v=TIAB99sEqzw.

www.ingramcontent.com/pod-product-compliance
Lightning Source LLC
Chambersburg PA
CBHW050807160726
48004CB00002B/735